WHAT DO YOU
KNOW ABOUT
ASTHMA?

What Do You Know About Asthma?

Martina Chukwuma-Ezike

To order additional copies of this book, contact:
Xlibris Corporation
800-056-3182
www.Xlibrispublishing.co.uk
Orders@Xlibrispublishing.co.uk
306457

Contents

DEDICATION

To all who have lost their lives to asthma

ACKNOWLEDGEMENTS

Marrying my husband is the best decision I have ever made in my entire life. He is a great inspirer, adviser, and motivator. He made me believe more in my capabilities. Thank you very much, Uchenna, for your love and support. I love you and our adorable daughter Pearl.

I wish my heart could say in words the love and respect I have for Ambassador Soni Abang. My father, brother, and best friend, I wouldn't be where I am today without him. Thank you for giving my life a definition.

To my brother Nnamdi, for all the times you have given, shared, listened; I am fortunate to have the world's best brother. I am very grateful. I want to specially thank my family, in-laws, friends, and colleagues, especially Rima for her love and support.

My sincere gratitude goes to the Lord Provost of Aberdeen, Councillor George Adam, Dr Mike Okiro, Inspector General of Police (Rtd), my mentor Dr Ian Small, Chairman Primary Care Respiratory Society for the UK, Monica Fletcher, Chief Executive Education for Health, Very Rev. Richard Kilgour, Senator Bassey Otu, Mr Garry Hunter, Mr. Oru, Mrs Liz Gillies, Pastor Chris Gbenle, and Pastor Wilfred Emmanuel.

I would like to say a big thank you to Dr Russell Williams, Dr Ian Heywood, and Nicki Duncan, Graduate Business School, University of Aberdeen, Dr Bryan Brook, Mrs Sonia Hudson, Mr Paul Doney, Mr Rod McDermid, Dr C. Okoye, Dr O. Oliyide, Dr O. Matthews, Dr J. Okuneye, and Mr Ogbonna Ukuku.

FOREWORD

Years ago, asthma was a debilitating condition which, in many cases, seriously limited what a person could do. As a result of greater knowledge about asthma and its treatment options, the ability to manage this disease has vastly improved over the years.

When you manage your asthma, you can do almost anything you want to do. Throughout this book, you'll learn how to keep your asthma well-controlled so that you too can continue to lead a healthy and fulfilling life.

This brilliant book is written for asthma sufferers, their families, friends and anyone who want to have a better understanding of asthma. Whilst this book is not intended as a substitute for consultation with health-care providers, it certainly does provide excellent first-hand guidance as to what those affected can do to prevent or control symptoms to enable them live healthy lives.

This beautifully written book is unique because it is sharp, brisk, and simple for anyone to read and understand. It will leave you with a lingering memory long after the book is closed.

The Trustees of Asthma and Allergy Foundation

INTRODUCTION

Living with asthma can be a frightening and unpredictable experience. Asthma can be life-threatening and difficult to manage if not properly understood. Most asthma deaths are preventable, and lots of people who have lost their lives to asthma would have been alive had they known they could effectively manage their symptoms and keep their asthma well-controlled.

If you have asthma, or if you are a parent, relative, friend, carer, or colleague of someone with asthma, you will find the information contained in this book very helpful.

This book provides practical information that will help people with asthma manage their symptoms to enable them to live an active, healthy, and symptoms-free life and not living lives compromised by their asthma. It emphasises the importance of self-management since the responsibility for the day-to-day care rests entirely on people living with asthma and their families.

Results from recent research on asthma have emphasised the essential role of self-education. This book *What Do You Know About Asthma* focuses on the importance of patient education in the management of asthma because the more informed a patient is, the better they would be at managing their symptoms and keeping it under control.

Chapter 1 begins with the definition of asthma, indicating its symptoms and triggers, while Chapter 2 focuses on diagnosis, which involves medical and family histories, physical examination, and lung function among other tests. Chapter 3 explores the different classifications of asthma, ranging from mild to severe persistent asthma. Chapter 4 contains a discussion of different measures used in controlling the illness since asthma has no cure. It also looks at the various treatment options available. Chapter 5 and 6 provide information on the importance of control, how to achieve effective control of the disease, and what you can do to take care of your asthma. Chapter 7 looks at the major concerns people have, especially during pregnancy, while travelling, and when seeking employment. Chapter 8 explains what happens during an asthma attack and what you can do to help someone who is having an asthma attack. The final chapter explores the numerous myths surrounding asthma.

In writing this book, I contacted many sufferers who generously provided feedback alongside the questionnaires, shading more light on their personal experience of living with the condition, so I could learn from them while trying to make a difference by putting this text together. Also, knowledge gained from many years of working with people with asthma, other literature and my personal experience as an asthma sufferer.

CHAPTER 1

What is Asthma?

Have you, or your relative, been diagnosed with asthma? If yes, lots of questions will be running through your mind. You may be wondering as to what exactly is asthma, what causes it, and how it can be treated or cured.

Asthma has been defined as a disease that causes chronic inflammation of the airways -a tiny passage by which air reaches the lungs. Asthma is believed to be a serious lung disease. Asthma can affect anyone, and as a chronic disease, it needs to be monitored and controlled over a lifetime.

The cause of asthma is not yet known, and currently, there is no cure. Though asthma has no cure, countless people with asthma have learned to live well through education, correct treatment, advice, and support. If you are one of the millions of people with asthma, you too can.

According to recent estimates, asthma affects 300 million people in the world; more than 25 million people in the United States have asthma, and about 5.4 million people in the United Kingdom are currently being treated for asthma. Although people of all ages suffer from the disease, it most often starts in childhood, currently affecting about 7 million children in the United States and about 1.1 million children in the United Kingdom. It is believed that asthma kills about 255,000 people worldwide every year.

To have a clear understanding of asthma, it is important to know how the airways work. The airways are small tubes that carry air in and out of the lungs. People who do not have asthma have normal airways. People with asthma have airways that are consistently swollen to some degree, and their airways are very sensitive.

Once any substance that irritates the airways is inhaled, they tend to react very strongly. When the airways react, the muscles around them tighten; this constricts the airways, causing less air to flow into the lungs. The swelling can also worsen, making the airways even more constricted. This will result in the airways forming more mucus than usual, and this will further reduce the size of the airways, making breathing more difficult.

Sometimes, asthma symptoms are mild and can disappear on their own or after minimal treatment with asthma medication. Sometimes, symptoms may persist and even get worse. When symptoms get worse, it may result to an asthma attack that will require emergency care. Asthma has no cure. Even when the symptom improves, or you feel completely well, you still have the disease, and it can resurface at any time. That is why it is important to always take medication as directed by a doctor even when symptoms disappear.

With proper treatment, most people with asthma are able to manage their symptoms. As a result, they have few or no symptoms, and they can live normal, healthy lives and sleep through the night with no disruption from asthma.

i. What causes asthma?

Anyone can develop asthma at any age, and there is no known specific cause of asthma. Although most researchers believe that some genetic and environmental factors interact to cause asthma, mostly in early childhood. These factors are:

- an inherited tendency to develop allergies known as atopy
- parents who have asthma
- certain respiratory infections during childhood
- contact with some airborne allergens or exposure to some viral infections in infancy or in early childhood when the immune system is developing.

Also, children who have low birth weight or are exposed to tobacco smoke can develop asthma. Tobacco smoke has been linked to a higher risk of asthma and also a higher risk of death due to asthma, wheezing, and respiratory infections.

Children of mothers who smoke and people exposed to second-hand smoke have a higher tendency of developing asthma. It is also believed that a good number of people who have hay fever (allergic rhinitis) also develop asthma; allergic reactions triggered by antibodies in the blood often lead to airway inflammation that is associated with asthma.

If asthma runs in your family, exposure to irritants might make your airways more reactive to substances in the air, for example, tobacco smoke. It is important to note that some factors might be more likely to cause asthma in certain people than in others.

You may have increased chances of developing asthma if you have a history of wheezing, even though you did not have a cold, eczema, or an allergic skin condition and inflammation in the nose, known as allergic rhinitis.

ii. What are the symptoms of asthma?

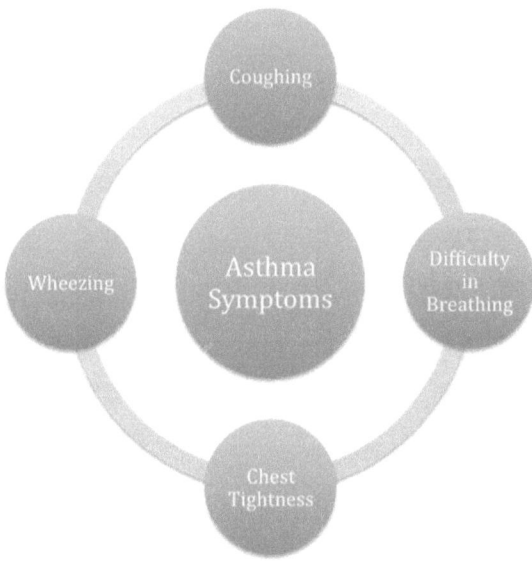

Asthma Symptoms

Asthma symptoms vary; you may have either all the symptoms or only some of them. Asthma symptoms may come and go. You may find you have symptoms at different times of the day; symptoms are often worse at night and at early hours of the morning. You may also have symptoms at different times of the year. Symptoms can be mild or severe, and the severity of asthma symptoms also varies from individual to individual. These symptoms include the following:

- difficulty in breathing
- wheezing—a whistling noise when you breathe
- chest tightness—the feeling that someone is squeezing or sitting on your chest
- faster or noisy breathing
- coughing

You may find out there are things that make your asthma worse. They are called asthma triggers.

iii. Asthma triggers

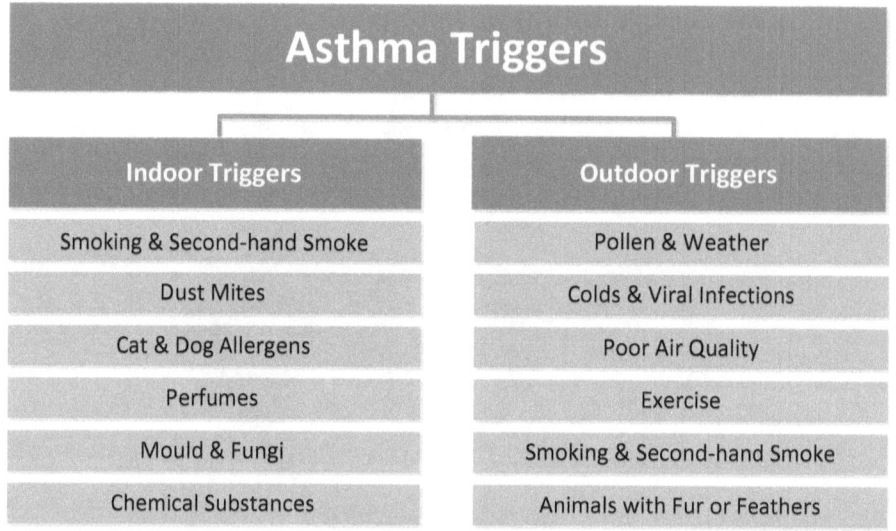

Asthma Triggers

Asthma trigger is anything that irritates your airways and causes asthma symptoms. Everyone has different asthma triggers, and most people have more than one asthma trigger. It is important to find out what your triggers are because if you can avoid or reduce your exposure to these triggers, you can get better control of your asthma.

While it is difficult to tell exactly what triggers someone's asthma, in some cases, the link may be clear, for instance, when your asthma symptoms start within minutes of inhaling dust or fumes from exhaust pipe. However, some people may have a delayed reaction to a trigger; in that case, the person will have to be very observant and possibly keep a record of the times when their symptoms got worse. Doing so will help identify what triggers your asthma. Asthma triggers could be indoor or outdoor.

Indoor asthma triggers: Indoor asthma triggers include inhaled allergens such as-smoking and second-hand smoke, dust mites, cat and dog allergens, perfumes, mould and fungi, chemical substances.

There are so many things you can do to help reduce triggers in your home; for example, not allowing anyone to smoke inside your home because tobacco smoke can irritate the airways and cause asthma symptoms. If you smoke, your doctor, nurse, or local pharmacy can offer advice and support on how you can quit.

Also, symptoms brought on by dust mites may be reduced by using barrier covers on your mattress, duvet, and pillows, using a damp cloth to dust, cleaning soft furnishings with anti-dust mite chemicals, removing all carpets and replacing with hard flooring, washing your sheets, duvet covers, and pillowcases with a hot temperature once a week, and vacuuming often (do ask someone to vacuum while you stay outside).

To avoid cat and dog allergens, it is advisable not to keep pets with fur or feathers. If you have pets, try to keep them away from your living room and bedroom, and bathe them regularly. If strong fragrances or scents from perfume or aftershave brings on your asthma symptoms, it is best for you not to use them. It will also be advisable to explain this to people you see often, asking them not to wear strong scents when you are together.

For mould and fungi, try to treat any damp as soon as possible, for example, using dehumidifier can help reduce damp. Keeping your home well-ventilated may also help reduce mould. Also, chemical substances kept at home or place of work can trigger asthma. Try not to keep chemicals at home, and for chemical substances at the place of work, make sure you discuss with the health and safety adviser and also see your doctor and asthma nurse as well.

Outdoor asthma triggers: Outdoor asthma triggers include pollen, weather, poor air quality from traffic fumes and pollution, exercise, colds and viral infections, smoking and second-hand smoke, animals with fur or feathers.

The following advice may help you avoid asthma triggers when you are out and about. To avoid contact with pollen, look out for pollen forecasts on the television, newspaper, or Internet. If pollen counts are high, try to reduce the time you spend outdoors. You may speak with your doctor or asthma nurse and seek advice on taking hay fever medication. A sudden change in temperature, cold air, windy and hot humid days can all cause asthma symptoms. Also, poor air quality may bring on asthma symptoms, so try not to stay out for too long or exercise outdoors during hot, sunny, or smoggy days.

Exercise is good for everyone, including people with asthma; however, some people have exercise-induced asthma. If you fall into this category, the following advice may be helpful. Always warm up before exercise and warm down afterwards; use your reliever inhaler before you exercise, and if you notice asthma symptoms during exercise, stop, take your reliever inhaler, and wait for sometime before starting again.

Also, colds and viral infections are very common asthma triggers and are almost impossible to avoid. Endeavour to take your flu vaccination to avoid any infection. If animals, smoke, and second-hand smoke triggers your asthma, try to avoid getting in contact with animals with fur or feathers and places where people smoke. Strong emotional expressions such as crying or laughing hard, cockroaches, and drugs such as aspirin and beta-blockers can also cause asthma symptoms.

When someone with asthma comes into contact with a trigger, the muscle around the walls of their airways tightens, their airways become swollen or inflamed, and sticky mucus builds up; this leads to asthma symptoms, and if nothing is done, it may lead to an asthma attack.

iv. Conditions linked to asthma

There are many conditions that are linked to asthma. They include the following:

Asthma and allergies: Most people with asthma also have allergies, although not everyone with allergies develop asthma and not everyone who has asthma has allergies. People are not born with allergies, but they may have genetic tendencies to develop allergies. It is believed that if both parents have allergies, there is a greater chance of their children developing allergies. Asthma and allergies, though related, have different meanings. While asthma is a disease that causes chronic inflammation of the airways, an allergy is a reaction of the body's immune system to substances that are usually harmless.

The human body reacts to anything perceived to be a threat; these substances do not cause any problem in most people, but once people with allergies come in contact with these substances, their immune system sees them as threats and reacts as a result. These substances are known as allergens; they can be inhaled, touched, swallowed, or injected. Some examples of allergens are mould, dust, pollen, and animal furs or feathers. Once exposed to allergens, they will have irritation or swelling in specific parts of their bodies like the skin, eyes, nose, and lungs. These allergens can make asthma symptoms worse by increasing the swelling in the airways and making them more sensitive.

Rhinitis and sinusitis: Though different, rhinitis and sinusitis are related conditions that can make asthma symptoms worse. Rhinitis is an inflammation of the inside of the nose caused by an allergen like dust, mould, pollen and so on. Rhinitis usually causes cold-like symptoms such as sneezing, itchiness, or blocked or runny nose. Sinusitis is when the lining of the sinus cavities become inflamed or infected; this happens as a result of viral, fungal, or bacterial infection. When someone with asthma develops rhinitis or sinusitis, it is important to see a doctor to receive appropriate treatments. Managing your rhinitis or sinusitis will help you have better control of your asthma.

Gastroesophageal reflux disease: Gastroesophageal reflux disease is also known as acid reflux, which, to most people, is ordinary heartburn. Acid reflux does bring on asthma symptoms in some people, for example, during coughing or when stomach acid travels up the esophagus and irritates the airways. If you suspect your asthma symptoms are caused by heartburn, make an appointment to see your doctor to have you checked for acid reflux.

CHAPTER 2

Diagnosing Asthma

Asthma is diagnosed based on medical and family histories, physical examination, and other tests. It is important that a doctor confirms you have asthma before you start any asthma treatment, the reason being that other conditions have similar symptoms to asthma, but asthma medicines would not be suitable for them.

i. Medical and family histories

Your doctor will ask if you have asthma symptoms, what symptoms you have, when and how often they occur. Your doctor will also ask if your symptoms get worse at night or early hours of the morning or when you exercise and what it is that triggers your asthma. Your doctor may also ask questions like whether you have any history of allergies like hay fever or eczema or if anyone else in your family has asthma or known allergies such as eczema, hay fever, or food allergies.

ii. Physical examination

Your doctor will listen to your chest and look for signs such as wheezing, swollen nasal passages, and allergic conditions like eczema. Note that you can still have asthma even if these symptoms are not present when your doctor carries out the examination.

iii. Lung function test

Measurement of lung function is used for the diagnosis of asthma as well as monitoring the course of the disease and the level of control. These tests include peak flow meter and spirometry. Peak flow meter is a device that measures how much air you can blow out of your lungs. Peak flow reading is an effective method used by most patients and their health-care providers to monitor asthma and evaluate the patient's response to therapy. Spirometry measures how well your lungs work. It measures the speed and amount of air you can blow out.

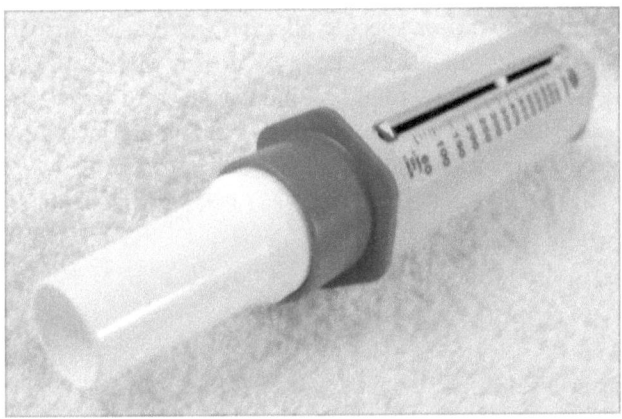

Peak Flow Meter

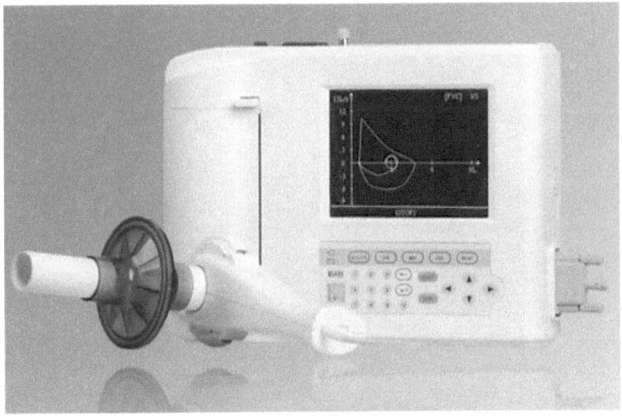

Spirometer

iv. Other tests

Other tests include reversibility test which measures your peak flow before and after you use reliever inhaler, a preventer, or steroids tablets. While exercise test measures your peak flow before and after a number of minor exercises. Sometimes, you may be offered a trial treatment to determine which inhaler will work best for you. The treatment your doctor prescribes will depend on the severity of your asthma.

Your doctor may also ask for other tests to be done, which include x-ray and lab tests on your blood and sputum. Your doctor may also refer you to an allergist who will test you for specific allergies, ask you what your symptoms are, and at what time you usually have or notice them. Allergists use skin prick test to find out what allergies make your asthma worse. Challenge tests can also be done in the hospital to help your doctor find out how hyper-responsive your airways are.

CHAPTER 3

Categories of Asthma

Asthma affects people differently; while some people may have mild asthma symptoms, others may have very severe asthma symptoms. Asthma has been categorised based on the severity of symptoms. The following are the categories of asthma, and this is based on when the sufferer is not taking any medications.

It is important to know that anyone with asthma can have a severe attack, even people with mild asthma.

i. Mild asthma

People with mild asthma have symptoms that come and go. These symptoms may manifest twice a week or less and are not disturbed by symptoms at night. Also, in-between asthma episodes, they have no symptoms, their lungs functions normally, and they can carry out their daily activities with no restriction.

ii. Mild persistent asthma

These categories of asthmatics have symptoms more than twice a week but not more than once in a day. They are usually awakened at night by their asthma, and this happens more than twice a month. They have asthma attacks that affect their activities.

iii. Moderate asthma

People with moderate asthma have symptoms every day, and they are usually bothered by nighttime symptoms at least once a week or more. Asthma attacks may affect their daily activities.

iv. Severe asthma

People with severe asthma have symptoms throughout the day; these could be most days of the week, and they hardly sleep through the night without being awoken by their asthma. Their asthma may also affect their physical activities, ranging from work, school, business, or other endeavours.

CHAPTER 4

Treatments

Asthma is a long-term disease that has no cure. The aim of asthma treatment is to effectively control the disease. With proper treatment, people with asthma can maintain good asthma control that will enable them to live a healthy, active, and symptoms-free life.

Your doctor will give you medications that will help control your asthma. With the right medicines, you should not have troublesome symptoms such as coughing and shortness of breath, asthma symptoms throughout the day, waking up at night because of your asthma, having asthma attacks, and needing to take your reliever inhaler. Taking the right medications also means your asthma will not interfere with your daily activities and help you maintain a good lung function, that is, your peak flow and spirometry readings will be normal.

The following are medicines that can help control your asthma. Your doctor will consider many things when deciding which asthma medicines are best for you. Your doctor will check to see how well a medicine works for you, after which he or she will adjust the dose as needed. Your doctor or asthma nurse should have offered you a written personal asthma action plan that will tell you when to take your medications, how much to take, and when to increase or reduce your dosage. Most asthma medicines are inhaled straight into the lungs, which makes them very effective.

i. Inhalers

There are two main inhaler medicines-relievers and preventers. All asthmatics should have a reliever inhaler (usually blue in colour); they are expected to take it once they have symptoms, and they should carry the inhaler with them at all times. Relievers are important in treating asthma attacks. Preventers are medicines that control the swelling and inflammation of the airways that make breathing difficult. They are usually brown, orange, or red in colour. They help reduce the risk of severe asthma attacks, and it is important you take them daily even when you do not have symptoms. Some people may be offered a combination inhaler; this inhaler acts as both preventer and reliever.

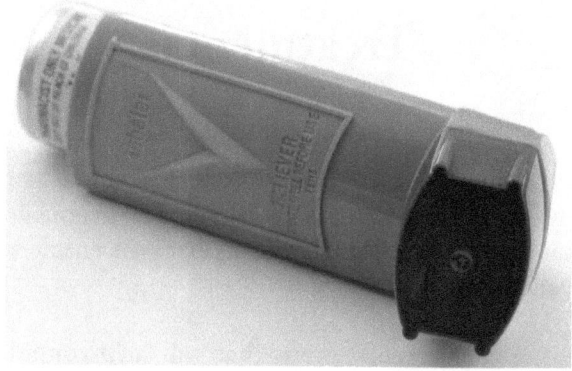

Reliever Inhaler

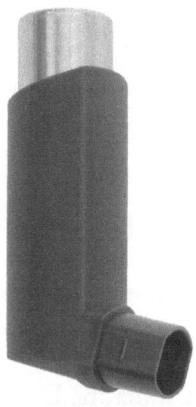

Preventer Inhaler

ii. Spacers

A spacer is a plastic or metal container with a mouthpiece at one end and a hole for the aerosol inhaler at the other. They only work with an aerosol inhaler. Spacers are very important because they help deliver the medicine straight to your lungs and also make it easier to use the inhaler.

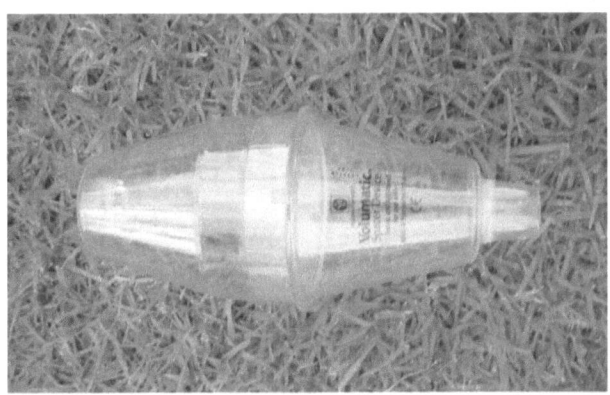

Spacer

iii. Corticosteroids

These are steroids used in treating asthma. They are made up of inhalers and tablets. These are very safe to take because our bodies produce them and are very different from those used by athletes. Inhaled steroids have side effects ranging from sore tongue and throat, a mouth infection known as thrush. It is recommended you rinse your mouth after using your inhaler to avoid these side effects. Also, the use of spacers can reduce the effect of getting thrush. Steroids tablets contain greater amounts of corticosteroids than preventer inhalers. Some people need to take short doses of steroids tablets to control asthma since they work faster to reduce inflammation. Others need to take steroids tablets for longer to help control their asthma.

iv. Other medicines

Other medicines used in treating asthma includes leukotriene receptor antagonists, which work by blocking one of the chemicals that is released when you come into contact with an asthma trigger; this medicine is steroids free.

Another medicine used in treating asthma is theophylline, which can be taken as a tablet, syrup, or an injection to help relax the muscles that surround your airways, making it easier to breathe, and does not contain steroids. Also, there are reliever tablets which work by opening up your airways by relaxing the muscles that surround them; these tablets do not contain steroids.

v. Emergency care

In more severe asthma attacks, lifesaving treatments will be administered at the hospital, and this includes oxygen which will be given through a mask if your oxygen levels are low. You will be given reliever medicine either through a drip or nebulizer. A nebulizer creates a mist of medicine which you breathe in through a mask.

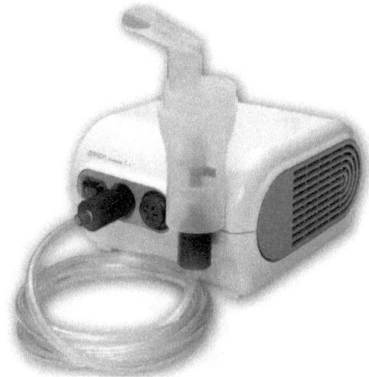

Nebulizer

While at the hospital, you may be given magnesium sulphate through a drip if you have life-threatening asthma or if other medicines don't work after you have had a severe asthma attack. Also, your specialist may give you aminophylline through a drip to treat severe asthma attack.

CHAPTER 5

Asthma Control

Learning as much as possible about asthma will help you to manage the condition properly. Asthma cannot be cured; however, there are steps that can be taken to control the disease and prevent its symptoms. Asthma that is not well-controlled can cause many problems, ranging from sleeplessness, not able to go to school or work, hospitalisation, and even death. However, with good asthma control, these problems are preventable.

To achieve this goal, ask your doctor about common asthma triggers. Your doctor will advise you and may refer you to a specialist or an asthma educator. To find out about your allergic triggers, your doctor will refer you to a specialist to carry out an allergy assessment. To identify non-allergic triggers, you may need to keep a diary of your symptoms. Once you know things that make your asthma worse, you can learn how to avoid them. To achieve and maintain total control of your asthma, you will need to take your medication as prescribed by your doctor, stay away from anything that makes your asthma worse, watch for signs that your asthma is getting worse and see your doctor as soon as possible, and keep regular check-ups or reviews for your asthma as well as asthma education.

i. Peak flow meter

In addition to the above, your doctor may suggest you use a peak flow meter to monitor your lung function. This will help you identify any changes that indicate your asthma is not well-controlled. Your doctor will also suggest you keep a diary of the results of your peak flow readings and symptoms so that both you and your doctor can use it to make a personal asthma action plan.

A peak flow is a simple device that measures your peak expiratory flow. Using a peak flow meter can help determine whether your peak flows vary over time or are affected by the presence of certain triggers. It can also monitor how well your medications are working, develop an asthma action plan, and determine if you require urgent medical attention.

To use a peak flow meter, simply read the instructions that come with the model that you have and do the following:

- Attach the mouthpiece to the peak flow monitor
- Set the marker or indicator to zero on the scale
- Stand up; if you cannot stand, try and sit upright,
- Take a deep breath, close your lips tightly around the mouthpiece
- Blow out as hard and as fast as you can
- Take note of the number close to the marker.
- Repeat the above steps up to three times; record the highest of the three numbers in your diary. This number signifies your peak expiratory flow.

Your doctor or asthma nurse will help you find out which of your peak expiratory flow measurements should be used as your best peak flow. Use your peak flow result with your written action plan to help you understand what you should do to manage your asthma. If your best peak flow is less than eighty per cent, it means your asthma is not well-controlled; ensure you discuss your results with your doctor. Apart from using your peak flow meter, it is important you monitor your symptoms to ensure your asthma is well-controlled.

ii. Signs that your asthma is not well-controlled

If your asthma is not well-controlled, there are signs you should not ignore. They are as follows: Your asthma symptoms are worse than what they used to be, you have symptoms more often than usual, you are awoken at night because of your asthma, you are unable to go to work or school because of your asthma, you have low peak flow reading, your asthma medication doesn't seem to work as it should, you are making use of your reliever inhaler more often, and you require emergency care because of an asthma attack or are admitted in hospital because of your asthma. Once you notice your asthma is getting worse, ensure you seek medical help as soon as possible because it may be that your asthma medicines need to be changed, and your doctor may take other steps to ensure your asthma is under control.

iii. Good asthma control

Good asthma control means that someone with asthma has no or minimal asthma symptoms, are not awoken at night by their asthma, no or minimal need to use their reliever inhaler, are able to do normal daily activities and exercise, no or very infrequent asthma attacks, and good lung function tests. Having good asthma control helps reduce the risk of having an asthma attack.

iv. Factors limiting good asthma control

There are many factors that limit good asthma control, and they vary from one country to another. The following are the most common factors.

Diagnosis: In some countries, for example, West Africa, most people with asthma may never receive a diagnosis and, therefore, will not have the opportunity to be given good or proper asthma treatment. Factors such as poor access to medical care, improper or lack of correct diagnosis by health practitioners, lack of awareness among sufferers as well as mistaking asthma symptoms for those of other diseases.

Treatment: Lack of access to medical care is one of the major factors that limit asthma control. Because of lack of access to hospitals and high cost of medication, most people with asthma cannot afford to go to big cities where hospitals are located, and the very few who go to hospitals cannot keep up with the recommended dosage; their asthma may not be well-controlled as a result. Also, asthma medications are not available in some areas such as West Africa, Middle East, Southern Asia and so forth.

Education: The level of asthma awareness in most countries is still very poor; for instance, in some parts of Africa, majority of the population do not know what asthma is, and they often attribute asthma to spiritual attacks or that the individual is possessed. Also, most people with asthma do not know how to use their medication correctly, and there are lots of misconceptions surrounding asthma treatments.

Environmental factors: The most effective way to reduce asthma symptoms and gain control is to stay away from triggers. However, in most countries, for example, in Africa, people with asthma are exposed to triggers such as pollution, dust from deplorable and untarred roads, poor air quality, smoke from a burning bush, stoves and firewood used in cooking, and chemicals in their places of work since there is currently no legislation or health and safety regulations to protect asthma sufferers.

Chapter 6

Living with Asthma

If you have asthma, it is important you learn how to take care of yourself. Here are some things you can do to help keep your asthma well-controlled.

i. Self care

Self-care is an important part of daily life. It means taking responsibility for your own health and well-being while getting support from those involved in your care such as doctors, nurses, carers and so forth.

ii. Take your medication

It is important you take asthma medicines exactly as your doctor tells you even if you feel better. Taking your medication daily will keep your asthma under control and can help prevent asthma attack. If you experience any side effects when taking your medication, ensure you speak with your doctor.

iii. Regular reviews

Always have your asthma reviewed every six months by your doctor. Ensure you tell your doctor all he or she needs to know so he or she can give you all the help that you need.

iv. Avoid triggers

Stay away from things that make your asthma worse. Also, watch for signs that suggest your asthma is getting worse and ensure you see your doctor as soon as possible.

v. Stop smoking

If you smoke, your doctor, nurse, or local pharmacist can offer advice and support on how you can give up smoking. Smoking reduces the effectiveness of asthma medication; quitting will significantly reduce the severity and frequency of symptoms. Also, if you do not smoke, avoid being exposed to tobacco smoke.

vi. Asthma action plan

Ensure you have a personal asthma action plan, which is usually a written information provided by your doctor or asthma nurse to help you understand more about your asthma and how to keep it under control.

vii. Peak flow meters and maintaining diaries

Perform peak flow meter testing, and keep a record of your measurement in your peak flow diary. (A peak flow meter is a small plastic tube used in measuring long function of people with asthma. Peak flow measurements allow you to see if your asthma is under control. Peak flow diary helps you to keep a record of your peak flow measurement).

viii. Inhaler technique

Ask your doctor or asthma nurse to teach you how to use your inhaler. This is very important because if you do not use your inhaler correctly, less medication will get into your airways, and you will end up having less medication.

ix. Exercise

Exercise is good for everyone, including people with asthma; however, some people have exercise-induced asthma. If you fall into this category, the following advice may be helpful. Always warm up before exercise and warm down afterwards; use your reliever inhaler before you exercise, and if you notice asthma symptoms during exercise, then stop, take your reliever inhaler, and wait for sometime before starting again.

CHAPTER 7

Asthma Concerns

i. Asthma and pregnancy-breathing for two

Once you find out you are pregnant, it is very important you look after your asthma because you will be breathing not only for yourself but also for your baby. Living well with your asthma means you can provide the best protection for your unborn child.

During pregnancy, the body undergoes different changes and that can also affect your asthma. The effect of pregnancy on women with asthma is unpredictable. While some women will notice an improvement, others will experience worsening asthma symptoms, and some women will not see any change in their symptoms.

It is important you keep your asthma well-controlled to enable you to have a healthy pregnancy. Speak to your doctor and seek advice on how best you can manage your asthma, and inform your doctor or midwife if you notice a change in your symptoms. Keep taking your asthma medicines because they are completely safe. Develop an asthma action plan with your care givers: doctor, asthma nurse, and midwife. The asthma action plan will describe which medicines you need, when to take them, and what to do if your asthma becomes worse.

There is a significant chance that your asthma may get worse during pregnancy, so prevention is vital. Ensure you take your medications as directed by your doctor. Although it is believed that taking steroids for a long time when pregnant can increase the risk of having a baby with low birth weight, remember that the risk associated with having an asthma attack outweighs any risks associated with asthma medicines; speak to your doctor if you are worried. Proper asthma control is necessary for pregnant women in order to ensure a good supply of oxygen to the foetus. Having an asthma attack during pregnancy is an emergency; if you are having a severe asthma attack, you should be treated in hospital and given all the necessary support.

Most women often ask whether it is safe to breastfeed while taking steroids; it is safe to breastfeed because your inhaled steroids go straight down to the airways. Very little is absorbed into the rest of the body, so it will not affect your breast milk. It is also important to note that, asthma, like many allergic conditions, runs in the family. If both parents have asthma, the chances of your baby developing asthma are higher. However, the chances of a child developing asthma are higher if the mother is an asthma sufferer.

ii. Occupational asthma

Occupational asthma is being in a job that puts you in contact with substances that can cause asthma. Such substances include wood dust, latex, and dust from insects and animals or from flour and grains. Examples of such jobs are joinery, spray painting, working in a laboratory, and jobs which involve the use of gloves, for example, nursing.

If you develop adult-onset asthma or if, as a child, you had asthma and it resurfaces, your doctor should consider if substances at your place of work could be responsible for your asthma. Questions such as 'is your asthma better on days you are off work or on vacation' would be asked by your doctor to help determine if your asthma is caused by your place of work. If you answer yes to the above questions, your doctor will then carry out a full investigation to find out if you have occupational asthma.

Diagnosing occupational asthma can be difficult; your doctor may have to refer you to a specialist. For a specialist to confirm you have occupational asthma, you would be asked to measure your peak flow at different times of the day when you are home and also at work. If the peak flow reading taken at home is better than the one taken at work, it is likely your asthma is caused by your place of work.

Once your specialist confirms that your asthma is work-related, you would be advised to avoid substances that cause your asthma at work by discussing with your employer to either remove the substances or change your role to enable you work where you will not be exposed to substances that bring on your asthma.

iii. Travelling with asthma

Having asthma should not prevent you from travelling and enjoying your holidays. Making the necessary plans on time will enable you stay safe while you are away holidaying. The following things should be taken into consideration while making your travel plans: health check, asthma triggers, air travel, travel immunisation, and travel insurance.

CHAPTER 8

Asthma Attack

Once people with asthma come in contact with a trigger, their airways constrict, making breathing very difficult; if nothing is done to open up the airways, it would lead to an asthma attack. Asthma attacks go through the following three stages:

- The airways become irritated and react to triggers such as smoke, pollen, and dust
- The airways narrow or become smaller and start producing mucous which reduces the size of the airway
- The airway muscles tighten, making breathing more difficult.

i. Signs and symptoms

- coughing or wheezing more than usual or feeling more breathless or chest feels tight
- unable to breathe easily and so finding it difficult to talk, eat, or sleep
- having to use the reliever inhaler more often than usual and reliever inhaler unable to help reduce the symptoms
- decreased activity level
- pale blue lips or fingernails
- sweating, anxiety, or fear

To avoid having asthma attack, you have to avoid your triggers that bring on your asthma symptoms and always try to keep your asthma well-controlled.

Asthma that is not well-controlled can cause problems such as sleeplessness, inability to attend school, hospitalisation, or even death. But many of these problems are preventable once your asthma is well-controlled.

To have good control of your asthma, it is important you take your asthma inhalers and preventers, and if possible, try and stay away from things that make your asthma worse-triggers. With you doctor's help, you can control your asthma and become free of your symptoms most of the time. But your asthma does not go away even when your symptoms go away, so it is important you take your medication even when you no longer have symptoms.

ii. Asthma first aid

First Aid Guide for Asthma

Follow the steps below to help someone having an asthma attack

If the person does not have a reliever inhaler, call 999 for emergency assistance

Sit the person upright

- Be calm and try to reassure the person
- Do not leave the person alone

2. **Give medication**

- Shake the reliever inhaler (usually blue)
- Use a spacer if available

3. **Wait four minutes**

- If there is no improvement
- Give two puffs of reliever inhaler (one puff at a time) every two minutes, you can give up to ten puffs

4. **If there is still no improvement, call 999 for an ambulance**

- Tell the operator the person is having an asthma attack
- Keep giving two puffs of reliever inhaler every two minutes until help arrives

Even if the person feels better, ensure they see their doctor same day. Remember that any delay in getting medical help when you have severe asthma symptoms can mean suffering needlessly and even death. Follow your doctor's advice, take your medication and avoid your triggers to enable you have better control of your asthma.

Asthma and Allergy Foundation
www.aaf-un.org

CHAPTER 9

Asthma Myths

Despite the prevalence of asthma, there is very little knowledge about the disease. People have lots of misconceptions about asthma. Below is a list of common asthma myths.

i. Asthma is often imagined

Asthma is not imagined or faked. It occurs because people with asthma have airway inflammation and constriction of the bronchi and bronchioles in their lungs. Triggers such as exposure to tobacco smoke or wood smoke, breathing polluted air, inhaling other respiratory irritants such as perfumes or cleaning products, exposure to airway irritants at the workplace, breathing in allergy-causing substances (allergens) such as moulds, dust, or animal dander, an upper respiratory infection such as a cold, flu, sinusitis, or bronchitis, exposure to cold, dry weather, emotional excitement or stress, physical exertion, or exercise can all trigger an asthma attack.

ii. Asthma can be cured

Asthma is a lifelong condition that can be effectively managed, but there is no cure. Education and self-management skills go a long way in helping patients with asthma monitor and manage their condition on a daily basis.

iii. Asthma symptoms are the same for everyone with asthma

Asthma symptoms vary from one person to another, both in its severity and the type of treatment required.

iv. One only has asthma when he or she has difficulty in breathing

That you don't have symptoms does not mean your asthma has gone away. Daily control with anti-inflammatory medication is required to help keep your asthma well-controlled. If not treated, asthma can be very serious and life-threatening.

v. One only needs to take his or her medication when he or she has difficulty in breathing

The inflammation of the airways needs daily treatment with controller medication. Take your controller medication regularly as prescribed; the benefits far outweigh the risks.

vi. People with asthma should avoid sports and physical activities

Asthma should not stop anyone from participating in sports or physical activities. Many professional athletes have asthma but are able to compete and excel because they have learned to manage their asthma. If you have difficulty taking part in sports or physical activities, it may be that your asthma is not well-controlled. Consult with your GP to assess your asthma and determine a proper exercise regimen for you.

vii. Children do outgrow their asthma

Asthma is a lifelong condition that will always require attention. A child's asthma may get less severe as he or she gets older, but it can return at any time.

viii. Taking steroids will stunt a child's growth

Studies have proven that steroids do not alter normal growth in children. Asthma, if left untreated, can result in permanent lung damage and have adverse effect on normal growth patterns. You should work with your GP or asthma nurse to find the right medications for your child's asthma.

ix. One should stop taking his or her controller medication once he or she feels better

It is important you keep taking your medication even if you feel better. If you stop taking your medication, the airway inflammation that leads to attack may return. Always consult with your GP before you stop taking your medication.

x. Steroids will harm unborn children

Steroid controller medications are inhaled, not swallowed, which means they act locally where they are needed and are not absorbed throughout the body. Also, research has shown that they are safe to be taken even when pregnant.

xi. Asthma medicine is addictive

Asthma is a chronic long-term condition. People with asthma may always need to take medication, but it is not because they are addicted to the medication.

xii. Children with asthma should not participate in exercise and sports

Children need to play and exercise to be healthy. Children with asthma can play and take part in sport, but they need to take their medication before they exercise. It is also important that they warm up before exercise sessions and warm down afterwards.

xiii. Asthma is contagious

Asthma, like many allergic conditions, runs in the family. If both parents have asthma, the chances of your baby developing asthma are higher. The chances of a child developing asthma are higher if the mother is an asthma sufferer. If the father of a child has asthma, the chances of that child developing asthma are much lesser. However, most people in Africa have a firm belief that asthma is contagious.

I remember an incident that happened in 2011, when I visited Africa; I had an encounter which I wouldn't forget in a hurry. At exactly 11.48 a.m., I was driving into a church premises when I saw a crowd. Out of curiosity, I hurriedly parked my car and went by to have a look. On the floor was a lady who, according to some, was possessed or had epilepsy. As soon as I looked at her, I realised she was having an asthma attack. On impulse, I hurried to help her up, and like a chorus, most of them said, 'Don't touch her! She's got asthma, and it's contagious.' But I was like, no, asthma isn't contagious. It took a lot of courage before a guy joined me to help the lady to a sitting position while I got my car to take her to the nearest hospital. The woman could have been dead if I wasn't at the scene. Their misconception about asthma is largely because of lack of asthma education or awareness.

REFERENCES AND FURTHER READING

American Thoracic Society. Health effects of outdoor pollution. Committee of the Environmental and Occupational Health Assembly of the American Thoracic Society. *Am J Respir Crit Care Med* 1996; 153: 3-50.

British Thoracic Society. *The burden of lung disease: a statistics report from the British Thoracic Society*. 2nd ed. London: British Thoracic Society; 2006.

Broadfield E, McKeever TM, Scrivener S, Venn A, Lewis SA, Britton J. Increase in the prevalence of allergen skin sensitization in successive birth cohorts. *J Allergy Clin Immunol* 2002; 109: 969-74.

Brown C, Hennings J, Caress A, Partridge MR. Lay educators in asthma self-management: reflections on their training and experiences. *Patient Educ Couns* 2007; 68: 131-38.

Ehrlich RI, Weinberg EG, Volmink JA, Potter P. Risk factors for childhood asthma and wheezing: importance of maternal and household smoking. *Am J Resp Crit Care Med* 1996; 154: 681-88.

European Community Respiratory Health Survey. Variations in the prevalence of respiratory symptoms, self-reported asthma attacks, and use of asthma medication in the European Community Respiratory Health Survey (ECRHS). *Eur Respir J* 1996; 9: 687-95.

Lung and Asthma Information Agency. Trends in hospital admissions for asthma. Factsheet 96/2.

Managing asthma in adults—a booklet for patients and their families and carers. Scottish Intercollegiate Guidelines Network, December 2011.

Masoli M, Fabian D, Holt S, Beasley R; Global Initiative for Asthma (GINA) Program. The global burden of asthma: executive summary of the GINA Dissemination Committee report. *Allergy* 2004; 59(5): 469-78.

McKinley Health Center. *Handout on asthma.* University of Illinois, 2008.

National Asthma Campaign. Out in the open: a true picture of asthma in the United Kingdom today. *Asthma J* 2001; 6(Suppl): 3-14.

National Institutes of Health. Global initiative for asthma. Natl Heart Lung Blood Inst Publ No. 95-3659. Bethesda, MD: NHLBI 1995; 6.

Neri M, Spanevello A. Chronic bronchial asthma from challenge to treatment: epidemiology and social impact. *Thorax* 2000; 55: S57-8, 2013.

Netuveli G, Hurwitz B, Levy M, Fletcher M, Barnes G, Durham SR, Sheikh A. Ethnic variations in UK asthma frequency, morbidity, and health-service use: a systematic review and meta-analysis. *Lancet* 2005; 365(9456): 312-17.

Smith A, Partridge MR. Greater expectations? Findings from the National Asthma Campaign's representative study of the needs of people with asthma (NOPWA) in the UK. *Asthma J* 2000; 5(3): 106-7.

World Health Organisation. *WHO strategy for prevention and control of chronic respiratory diseases.* Geneva: World Health Organisation; 2002.

INDEX